Wake Up Hungry for Life Starting Tomorrow

Goodbye Food Cravings! Hello Moderation!

OANA PITICAR

2021

Dedication

This book is dedicated to my late grandfathers, Aurel and Filip, my great grandmother Irina, and my auntie Maria. You are deeply missed and loved.

It is dedicated to my wonderful grandmothers Eugenia and Aglaia. So much love and respect goes to you both.

I am dedicating this book to my parents as well. Dorina-Maria and Adrian, it's all thanks to you. I am forever grateful.

To my sister Camelia, my niece Carina and my brother Ionut-Adrian, you are all indispensable.

Acknowledgements

A big thank you to my amazing friends Thani, Lisa, Nicoleta, Alex, Emilija, and Elena. I thank you for supporting me and believing in me.

To DJ Thomas. Thank you for your input in this book. I am so grateful for you, you are wonderful.

About the Author

Oana Piticar is a Romanian model and actress. She moved to London in 2012 and has been living there ever since.

When she was young, she loved helping people and dreamed of becoming a doctor. Despite following a different path when she grew up, she knew there would be another way of impacting someone's health other than medicine.

Oana has always been aware of the value and healing that nutrition brings to our lives. She constantly inspires the people around her to change their eating habits and create the best version of themselves.

Her aim through this book is to introduce and implement a new perception regarding food and its benefits. Oana also wants to encourage us to love ourselves fully, as self-love is where it all begins.

Table of Contents

Introduction

What do you think of when you see the phrase 'You are what you eat'?

For some, you'll think of it as the setup for a joke about being a certain animal or eating an abstract concept. You might also go down the transubstantiation route if you're Catholic. Maybe you're old enough to remember it being part of the nutritional mantra for the 1960s hippie movement. Others will see it as a quick introduction to persuading you to join their new diet. And then there are some who will tune the phrase out without a second thought after seeing it so many times.

Whatever your reaction, whatever your answer, I ask you to consider its true meaning and how it affects you. For you see, it's not just about what you eat, but also *why* you eat.

'You are what you eat' is a handy, memorable phrase to describe the effect food has not only on your body but also on your mind. It's meant as both a cautionary tale and a teaching phrase. If you were to expand the phrase, you could say that *what you choose to eat will change you physically and mentally.*

Now, this might paint food in a bad light, and that's not the intention here. In fact, we're trying to accomplish the exact opposite here by painting food in the best light possible. Acclaimed therapist and best-selling author, Marisa Peer, provides an expanded, optimistic outlook on this phrase. She believes that what we "eat, think, and do" can be positive forces of change in our lives.

And really, what better outlook can you have on eating and food in general? Food is good. Food is great. Food is life just as much as it is life-changing!

Food is a gift that continues to give, we're constantly finding new ways to nourish our bodies whether it's through new spice combinations or studying the health benefits of certain ingredients. People study for years in order to turn food into works of art, pleasing to both your eye and your palette. When you give food to those who can't give back, it can be used to communicate trust or kind-heartedness. Food has literally connected the world through intercontinental trade routes, introducing new recipes and uses for ingredients in countries that they maybe never would have figured out on their own. Akin back to the spice trades from continent to continent and the certain cooking and food preservation methods passed down to foreigners visiting new places. Compare that to the potlucks we have now, and the fusion restaurants blending intercontinental cuisine; food has always, in some way, been a great communicator.

Food is a universal blessing, meant to be an inalienable right for anyone and everyone. Food literally gives you power: the power to function and process things throughout the day, the power to perform physical and mental feats, the power to be better than you were the day before.

You are what you eat, which means food becomes a part of your identity.

The problem comes when you turn food into your *whole* identity.

Especially now when food is in much more abundance than it has been throughout the centuries, we have given a worrying amount of control to the nutrition (or lack thereof) we put into our bodies. We scrap for certain kinds of food, disregard others entirely out of our diet due to the taste or inability to satisfy us, and unfortunately, we also eat much more than we should.

Overeating has caused us to give too much control to our food intake, keeping us from knowing when enough is enough. Unhealthy food cravings give control to certain kinds of food that are good in small doses, but not all the time. Just as unfortunate, if not more, are those who have an unhealthy relationship with food entirely, seeing it as an enemy that's keeping them from being fit and healthy.

This is not what food is supposed to be, and yet it is through this mindset we have developed over food, this is the harsh reality that we live in.

But there is a great bright spot to this, which is that this is *not* a permanent change. We are not doomed to food damnation. You are not shackled to have an unhealthy relationship with food forever. You can rise up from the muck in a way that requires no tools, no paid programs, and no outside help. Through a reshaping of your mind, a reflection on your relationship with food, and the implementation of certain techniques, you can take back control of your entire life and place food back in the role it's meant to be in.

And that, dear reader, is why this book exists. It is why you have decided to pick this up and read it and understand its worth to you. This book is designed to help you massively in taking back that control and building new healthy habits around food. Whether you are struggling with food cravings or overeating, or simply have a desire to be in a truly joyful relationship with food, this book is for you.

You are what you eat, so consider this book as food for thought, and when you wake up tomorrow, you won't be hungry for bad relationships or perceptions. You won't be hungry for food that won't enrich you or nourish you. You won't be hungry for the food you've been conditioned to want.

You'll be hungry for life.

Chapter One

Build a Healthy Relationship with Food

To determine why you've cultivated a negative mindset with food, you have to take an in-depth look at your relationship with food. What does it mean to you? Do you have a good relationship with food? Or a bad one? How can you even tell?

Let's look at some differences between a good relationship with food and a bad one.

Good vs. Bad Relationship with Food

We want to build a better, healthier relationship with food, so let's look at what a bad relationship looks like. That way we have a frame of reference, a comparison to go back to.

A bad relationship with food is characterized by resentment, guilt, shame, and a need for over-the-top control. If you're thinking too much about what you're eating and how much, those are initial signs of a bad relationship with food. It's almost as if food is a significant other that you don't fully trust. You're constantly looking out for them, wondering where they are and what they're doing, afraid of their responses to things you might say or do, and there's no love or enjoyment around them.

When you have a bad relationship with food, some of these still apply. You're constantly checking a calorie counter to figure out how much you're still allowed to eat that day, you're jumping on to one fad diet after another hoping that the next one will stick, you ignore your body's signals when you're actually hungry, you avoid and restrict foods that you've deemed "bad," and you just have this overall feeling of guilt toward eating.

It's not fun if you have a bad relationship with food, it's stressful and leads you down some bad paths. Left unchecked, it becomes the enemy of sorts that keeps you from living life to the fullest. When in reality, food is what's needed to help you feel fully alive.

Food, as we discussed in the introduction, is *good*. And your relationship with it should be good too.

A good relationship with food is classified by trust, freedom, and appreciation for it being more than just nutrition and sustenance. It takes time and patience to develop this kind of relationship, but it's very much worth it in the end.

When you have a good relationship with food, you enjoy what you like in moderation. It becomes less about what you're eating or how much, and more about what you like to eat and when. You don't concern yourself with this concept of good or bad foods, you eat what you like and eat until you're full. There is no overindulgence, guilt, or anxiety whenever you're eating, you love whatever's on your plate and that's that.

It's not about a diet, it's not about calorie counting, and it's not about what to eat and when. It's about you and how much you enjoy whatever you've made or what someone else has made for you.

But how do we get to that point? How do we better our relationship with food?

Five Tips To Better Your Relationship With Food

Canadian dietician Katey Davidson has done some extensive research on food relationships, and she developed these five tips that will help you wherever you're at with food (Davidson, 2020). Notice as you're reading through them how none of these tips have anything to do with what to eat or what not to eat. In fact, they barely police you on your intake at all. These tips draw from your mindset, not your diet.

1) **Unconditional Permission:** Don't set rules on what you're allowed to eat or when you're allowed to eat. Your body does not run on the clock that the world does; when it's hungry, it's hungry. If you restrict your food intake to a certain number of calories or certain foods, you can develop a fear of food. And when you restrict yourself to only eating at certain times of the day, your hunger and depravity increase. Give yourself the time and grace to eat whatever you want and whenever you want (within reason, of course). Remind yourself that you deserve to eat when you're hungry, and your body deserves food. Doing this will help give you a positive connotation toward food, you're able to embrace it rather than rejecting it.

2) **Eat When Hungry,** *Stop When Full:* Relating back to the first tip, you don't want to overindulge on food or stop eating way before your body's had its full. Did you ever grow up being told that you couldn't leave the table until you finished everything on your plate? Were you made to feel guilty over the mention of how hard your parents

worked on the meal? Were you lectured on the fact that there are children on the other side of the world who would love to eat all the food that's left on your plate? This guilt manifests later in life by making you believe that you're done eating when your plate's empty, which leads to both undereating *and* overeating. You don't listen when your body's full, you listen to the clean plate in front of you. On the other side of this extreme, you finish eating when you've reached some sort of caloric limit. Even if you're still hungry, you've allotted the recommended number of calories for this particular meal which means you're done.

This is not how it's meant to be. Listen closely to your body, specifically your stomach. If you are full, then stop eating right there, not before or after. This will help you better manage your food intake and get you more in-tune with your hunger pangs.

3) **Mindful Eating:** A mental wellness method that's been growing in popularity in recent years is mindfulness, which is the practice of getting rid of internal and external distractions and being in the present moment. It's useful in combating anxiety, racing thoughts, and low self-worth.

Mindfulness can also be used to better our relationship with food through the process of mindful eating. This is a little more involved than most mindfulness practices because it requires intentionally getting rid of not just internal distractions, but also outside distractions such as the TV or your phone. Your focus must be on the food in front of you and nothing else, that way you're able to savor the flavors, textures, sights, and smells. By intentionally and slowly eating, you learn to fully enjoy your food, you start asking yourself some much-needed questions.

Am I eating because I'm hungry or because I'm bored? Do I like this kind of food more than others? Am I eating to make myself feel better physically or mentally? Does this food satisfy a craving that I have? Once you open yourself up to these questions, you have a more intentional relationship with your food.

4) **Don't Exclude Food:** Note that this tip is not meant for those whose religion or body restricts them from eating certain foods. For example, if you can't eat meat because of your religion or you can't eat gluten because you have Celiac disease, then you can disregard this tip.

But for those who are voluntarily excluding foods or labeling them as 'bad' because of a diet they chose to go on, you are doing yourself a grave disservice. Not only are you reducing your palette to a few choice tastes, but your appetite for those 'restricted' foods grows immensely. This is especially true for foods that aren't nutritious but taste delicious like desserts and junk food.

Those who don't restrict themselves with these kinds of foods have been found to better regulate themselves while eating them, meaning they're much more capable of stopping their intake when they've had their fill. Those who keep from eating these foods will end up overeating when finally giving themselves their permission to indulge. This is known as counter-regulation.

5) **Don't Justify Yourself:** How many times have you said any form of this statement: "I have had a good day, so I think I'll treat myself to ___."

Why do you have to explain why you're eating what's on your plate? Isn't it enough just to say that you enjoy it and that's why you're eating it? And even if someone did ask why you're eating a certain food, you don't actually have to justify your choices to them. Give yourself the grace and freedom to eat whatever you feel like eating at that given time because when you start feeling guilty over your food choices, that's when you start making food the enemy.

Food is not the enemy here, no matter what kind of stigma surrounds certain foods and the shame we're meant to feel when eating. This chapter is especially important for you as a reader because it will set up your mindset for food going forward. Take a long, hard look at where food stands with you and figure out what it will take to have a better relationship with it. Because that relationship with food is the foundation on which every chapter will be built on.

Chapter Two

Mindless Eating Into Mindful Eating

There was a certain tip in the last chapter that needs to be further examined, and that is the practice of mindful eating. By examining your food choices and eating habits, you learn more about yourself and what you enjoy, thus finding more enjoyment in food. Before we dig further into this practice, we should look at the opposite practice of mindless eating.

What Is Mindless Eating?

To put it simply, mindless eating is distracted eating. It's any time that you eat where your focus is on anything other than the food that's in front of you. Your mind tends to make a lot of unconscious decisions throughout the day, which is good because it would be tedious reminding yourself every second to blink and breathe. One decision that shouldn't be unconscious is eating, it should not be a background process while you're focused on other things.

Mindless eating can take on many forms. These include sitting in front of the TV or using your phone while eating, emotional eating in order to feel comfort or assurance, eating when you're bored, or eating directly out of the bag or box that the food came from.

How To Stop Mindless Eating

Thankfully, it's much harder to identify mindless eating habits than it is to kick them. There are several things you can do to minimize and even eliminate mindless eating, which will help in your transition to mindful eating.

Retrain your mind using visual tricks and cues. By eating food on smaller plates and drinking out of taller glasses, it satisfies that 'clean plate' signal and allows us to feel full without eating so much. Bigger plates tend to make portions feel smaller, and smaller glasses tend to make you feel like you didn't drink as much as you actually did. Reshaping those perspectives helps you know how to better decide when enough is enough.

Another visual trick to use is limiting your variety of junk foods and candy. When faced with too many choices, we end up feeling overwhelmed and will eat more to not 'miss out' on the various choices available to us. By giving yourself fewer choices of junk food and candy, you become numb to the stimulus, causing you to eat less of what you have. This is called 'sensory-specific satiety'. And it's a very effective mind trick that you can use for other breakable habits outside of food.

Find ways to make you work for the food that you want to snack on. If you have a bowl of chocolates by your desk, there's more than a guarantee that you'll mindlessly pick through that throughout the day. But if you place that bowl in your kitchen or make it so that you have to construct whatever you feel like snacking on, you're less likely to overindulge. That's because it's too much of an inconvenience to satisfy a craving that won't last that long.

And of course, there is the suggestion in the last chapter of getting rid of visual and auditory distractions while eating. If you 'unplug' before eating, you're much less likely to overeat because you don't have a lengthy distraction like a TV show or YouTube video in front of you to eat with. When it's just you and your food, you'll realize you don't need to eat all that much or for as long as you think. Oddly enough, this tip also works when it comes to using the restroom as well.

What Is Mindful Eating?

Mindful eating is a technique that is influenced by a key, universal process of mindfulness. This is not a new psychological fad, it's an inherent action that our mind does which can strengthen us mentally and emotionally. There is definite proof of a positive correlation between mindfulness and a change in eating habits and food intake, and when you look at the function of mindfulness this makes perfect sense. Mindfulness grounds you in the present, and tasks you with understanding where your body and mind are at that moment, it's all about awareness. How much awareness do you give to your eating habits or how much food you eat? How many times do you 'listen to your stomach' whenever you feel like eating?

We define mindful eating as a non-judgmental awareness of how food makes us feel when we're eating it or in an environment where food is around. It is not about what you're eating, but why and how you're eating. Mindful eating allows us to understand our cravings and hunger pangs, reduces the stress and guilt from eating, and helps us in savoring the food that we're eating. It has been known to help with eating disorders along with the depression and anxiety that come with eating. Mindful eating engages all your senses, keeps you from eating quickly or with distractions, and helps you to notice what food does not just to your body but also to your mind.

Mindfulness alone can help with some of these aspects, and in fact, regular mindfulness tactics have shown to help facilitate or transition people into learning mindful eating tactics. But to give yourself the best chance at combating food and eating stigmas, we will focus specifically on mindful eating. And thankfully, there are more than enough techniques and tips to help **you learn this process.**

How To Start Mindful Eating

An easy tactic to begin your mindful eating journey is to learn how to eat slowly. This feels like a no-brainer, but when was the last time a meal without distractions took you longer than fifteen minutes to finish? Studies say that it takes around twenty minutes before you even begin to feel full during a meal, so if you want to learn what it means to be full then slow your pace down, chew your food thoroughly, and ensure that there are no distractions around you. Focus on the flavors and textures, how it makes you feel, what parts of the meal are your favorite, and anything else that's based on what you're eating. Not only does this help with savoring your food, but it gives your body time to slow down and process things, making mealtimes a more relaxing part of your day.

Speaking on the topic of distractions, it's important that nothing is in front of you other than the food you're eating. It's a common practice to watch something while eating. In fact, it's almost second nature at this point to pull out our phones while eating or taking our food from the kitchen to the living room or wherever the TV is. We don't think too much about it, and that's where the problem lies. There is a strong link between visual distractions and overeating because subconsciously we are eating at the pace of whatever we're watching. But since our focus is on what's on the screen, we don't pay attention to our chewing or food intake. When we 'miss-time' our meals with the runtime of the show or video, we compensate by grabbing more food beforehand or during the meal.

It's easier to shut down those distractions beforehand and much more beneficial to you and your body. Turn off the TV, put your phone down, and eat in silence. It might feel strange and uncomfortable at first, but as time goes on this feeling will fade. Combine this with the earlier tactic of slow, thoughtful eating. Fill that silence with introspection, consider the ingredients of your meal and how it's made, think about how the food makes you feel. Within that awareness, your enjoyment of your meal will increase.

Much like regular mindfulness calls us to be in tune with our emotions during certain situations in our everyday lives, mindful eating calls us to be in tune with our emotions during a meal. Before you even go to eat, take a second to check in with your body and ask yourself a simple question: Why do you want to eat? This is not about trying to justify your food choices; this is more about slowing down and being in tune with your body and mind.

Are you hungry or are you bored? Are you hungry or are you looking for a source of comfort? Are you hungry or are you avoiding something? Food is not meant to be an escape; it is comfort and nutrition. Do not substitute proper emotional confrontation with a chocolate bar. And if you're really honest with yourself, it's not that hard to figure out whether or not you're hungry because hunger affects our bodies and behavior so much.

Try these methods out for one meal to start off. For one meal, shut down and get rid of all distractions, chew slowly and deliberately, and think about how the food makes you feel and what makes it so enjoyable. It will feel strange at first, much like all new changes to our behavior, but it gets easier the longer you do it. And pretty soon, you'll be kicking bad eating habits, cutting down on emotional and distraction eating, and on the right track towards a healthier view of food.

Chapter Three

Combat Overeating

Overeating is one of those things that you don't tend to notice you're doing until you've been doing it for a while. And *if* you leave it unchecked for too long, overeating becomes a nasty habit too hard to break. Over time, this habit will result in you gaining weight and warping your perspective on food.

Marissa Peer has done a wonderful write-up on the effects of overeating, and even classifies certain types of overeaters to help us better understand why it is that people indulge more than they should. These types of overeaters include the addictive eater, which is when one has far too many cravings and eats far too quickly because they need the chemicals the food gives them more than the food itself, and the habitual eater, which is when one has been conditioned to eat when they see food and not when they're actually hungry. If these kinds of emotions and thought processes resonate with you in some way, chances are that you are an overeater. And if that's the case, then this chapter will be especially useful for you.

One major piece of advice that people give to combat overeating is to ensure that you eat 'everything in moderation'. This is a phrase that gets thrown around a lot that it's in danger of being overused, and it has also become an excuse for people to eat more than originally planned due to, ironically, a lack of moderation. This is something that differs for everybody depending on their body and the kind of food that they need, and the foods that people typically 'moderate' are junk foods and sweets. What might be enough food for you might not be enough for another person, and that vagueness brings about certain problems because there is no strict limit for a moderate level. If you're going to eat in moderation, work with a food intake level that's doable for you so you don't find yourself overindulging or undereating.

Is there more that one can do to combat overeating other than moderate their food intake? Of course! There is an abundance of tips and tricks to help kick this nasty habit. Noted dietician Jillian Kubala outlines several simple methods that can help. Note the similarities between some of these and the 'mindful eating' tips from the last chapter.

Twenty-One Simple Ways to Stop Overeating

Get rid of distractions while you're eating, save for when you're in a social situation where the meal is less important than the company.

Know which foods will trigger you to start overeating or snacking more than necessary. Then get rid of those foods or make them difficult to access.

Don't ban foods from your diet; marking something as forbidden actually makes them more enticing. And if you 'give in' to those forbidden foods, you tend to go overboard on eating them. Make room for all foods in your diet, even treats. This does *not* apply to those addicted to certain foods, where it is better to deprive yourself of that food and find a healthier substitute.

Consume low-calorie, high fiber foods like grapefruit, non-starchy vegetables, and beans before a meal to feel full and avoid overeating. This is a process called volumetrics.

Never eat straight out of the container. Portion out what you want to eat into a plate or bowl in order to control the amount of food you actually eat.

Reduce the stressors in your life as well as taking up practices to relieve stress. There is an unfortunate correlation between stress and overeating which we touched on in the last chapter. Popular stress relievers are listening to music, yoga, deep breathing exercises, and relaxing.

Food's rich in fiber have been found to satisfy cravings and keep you fuller for longer, helping with the urges not just to overeat but also to eat when you're not actually hungry. Examples of fiber-rich foods include nuts, oats, and fruit.

Eat throughout the day rather than skipping meals entirely, this helps reduce food intake and hunger pangs. Holding off on meals or refusing to eat during certain times of the day can cause you to overindulge when you finally decide to eat. Again, this does not apply to those skipping meals due to religious or medical reasons.

Track your food intake and eating times using a food journal, be it a written one or through a mobile app. This can not only help you understand what you eat on a regular basis, but also with identifying potential situations and emotional triggers that can cause you to overeat.

Eat with those who have similar dietary beliefs and health goals that you do. People are more inclined to eat certain types of food and in varying amounts based on those that they're eating with.

Protein is not only a necessary strength-building component in food, but it can also help keep you full and energized throughout the day. Start off the day with a high-protein breakfast such as eggs to stave off morning hunger pains, and add protein-rich foods into your diet like almonds, chicken, Greek yogurt, and broccoli.

High blood sugar levels are also known to increase hunger, so it's important to regulate your blood sugar by limiting the intake of sweets and white bread and introducing foods in your diet like brown rice and beans.

Eat slowly and savor your food. Eating too fast is a major link to overeating, and it also decreases your enjoyment of the meal and your ability to feel full afterward.

For those legally allowed to drink, limiting your alcohol intake can also help you from overeating. Avoid binge drinking, and either cut alcohol out entirely or limit yourself to one drink during a meal.

Keeping healthy snacks on hand, carrying around a water bottle, and preparing meals beforehand ensure that you're planned when real hunger strikes. Not being prepared for your hunger makes it easier for you to buy quick, unhealthy foods and to eat more than you should.

Drinks with high-sugar content like sodas and certain fruit juices make you hungrier and also put you at risk of sugar-related diseases like diabetes. Cut back or cut out sugary drinks from your diet and replace them with water.

Check yourself, consider your mood and thought processes when you feel like eating. Are you hungry or bored? Do you need food right now to satisfy your hunger or to fill a certain void?

Avoid currently popular diets as well as short-term, food-restrictive diets. While they can result in weight loss at first, they are not sustainable and you'll find yourself overindulging in the foods you kept away from after you consider your diet over. Which will just bring you back to where you started. Make changes to your diet that you can sustain in the long term or throughout the rest of your life. Diets should not have a timeframe.

Take the time to seriously think about any old, unhealthy eating habits you may have such as eating in front of the TV or eating ice cream after work. It's hard to kick habits, but understand that doing so will leave you better off in the long run. This tip is easier to facilitate if you've been keeping a food journal.

Foods that are high in fat are not the enemy, especially those high in healthy fats like avocados, seeds, and olive oil. Introducing high fats into your diet, along with lowering your carb intake, can leave you less hungry after a meal for a long time.

Understand why you're trying to change in the first place, let this become a motivating factor for you. Set short-term and long-term goals that you can look back on during this journey of yours. Writing these down and having them readily available can keep you on track.

Don't feel intimidated by such a long list. A lot of these steps complement each other, and some of them you might already be doing subconsciously. Don't feel intimidated in trying to do every single step either. Work with the steps that work for you, find the ones that you're comfortable with doing consistently. Take your time and give yourself a chance, and your overeating habit will become a thing of the past.

Chapter Four

How To Actually Love Yourself

Self-improvement of any kind stems from a want **to** become better than you already are. But in that wanting feeling, there exists an underlying motivation factor which can either be good or bad. In other words, our need for self-improvement comes from whether we hate ourselves or love ourselves. It's all about perspective, what we think of the person in the mirror shapes our decisions and thought processes throughout our lives.

If your self-improvement stems from strong self-hatred, it means that you look in the mirror and see everything that you're not and blame yourself for 'letting yourself go'. You want to be better than what you see in the mirror, but it's because you hate what you see. This dictates the attitude you have in your health journey and the steps you'll take during it.

You'll use a lot of negative self-talk like 'This isn't good enough' or 'I ate too much today, why am I like this?'. You'll engage in self-destructive behaviors like prolonged starvation, rapid weight-loss schemes, overexercising, and overindulging with the promise of getting back on track tomorrow. You'll see yourself less as a human and more as a test subject in constant need of evaluations and experiments, deeming yourself a failure when you don't get your desired results.

There are many things that we attribute to this kind of behavior such as 'tough love' and 'discipline', but these are just positive-sounding terms meant to keep from accepting the fact that we hate ourselves. Which is awful. Self-hatred is not how anyone should live, neither is it anyway someone should treat themselves. Our lives are a gift, our bodies are a gift. Who we are and who we choose to vary vastly from those around us, and that's what makes us so beautifully unique.

It's okay if you want to change things about the body that you came in, but you must do so because you love yourself. Change is important to you because you love yourself enough to make good changes and be better than you were the day before. You love yourself enough to know that you deserve better. You love yourself enough to be the best version of yourself. This is the kind of mindset we need to have if any of the advice in this book is going to work. We need to love ourselves so that we're capable of making the necessary choices to be healthier and happier.

But what does it mean to love yourself? It's a phrase in danger of not really meaning anything, especially since it feels like such a vague concept and much less tangible compared to hating yourself. Fortunately, it does have a meaning that's just as tangible. In this chapter, we will explore the concept of loving ourselves, what it ultimately means to you, and addressing certain ways to help you learn to love yourself.

This may seem like an irrelevant part of the book, but it's actually one of the most important points to consider and it's a pleasure to be speaking about it now.

What Does It Mean?

To love yourself has many interpretations but they all center around a universal meaning. Loving yourself means having the ability to look at who you are and be not just content with what you see, but proud of it. Loving yourself means that you hold your well-being in great regard and will go to lengths to ensure that someone is taking care of you, that your own needs are met. No one else will give you the amount of love you deserve to show yourself, and the second you accept that is the second you can start working towards a greater level of self-love.

Loving yourself does mean that you'll have to put yourself first sometimes, which might be uncomfortable for you, but it's necessary. It's a primary step in learning *how* to love yourself, much like learning how to crawl is a primary step before learning how to walk. But there are some fascinating benefits when you love yourself.

Most obviously, learning to love yourself will raise your self-esteem and self-worth due to the positivity and support you're bestowing on to yourself that you might have only bestowed onto others. That self-worth allows you to see things from a better perspective and you learn to recognize what relationships you have that aren't respecting that self-worth, helping you to break from those unhealthy and at times codependent relationships. Self-love also helps you be more comfortable with yourself and what you like about yourself, making it easier to change certain aspects of your life because you no longer see it as a shameful correction of failure but rather a betterment of your body and a need to take care of it.

That final benefit is the strongest correlation between this book and the concept of self-love. When you learn to love yourself, you have more grace and patience with yourself to make lifestyle changes like with your diet and your perception of food. When you slip up, you don't berate yourself for it and instead, you pick yourself back up and keep trying. When you make progress, you're more inclined to be proud rather than telling yourself it's not enough yet.

Learn To Love Yourself

This isn't some sort of shift in thinking or life-long endeavor. Self-love is a perfectly attainable goal with actual methods and practices to help you achieve it.

One of the most effective self-love methods is to learn how to be comfortable by yourself. There is a strange feeling of both uncomfortableness and insecurity when it comes to doing things by yourself, especially in social settings like restaurants and movie theaters. But like it or not, the person you're going to spend the most time with in life is yourself. So why not make that alone time enjoyable? Become one of your own best friends, do fun things alone like going to the movies or the mall, treat yourself the way you would treat those you care about.

Alternatively, give yourself the grace to rest and take some downtime. After a long, busy week, relax your mind and body with some much-needed rest at home or by doing something fun that you don't need to prepare. Doing things for yourself can be exhilarating and cathartic, and if you can enjoy doing things on your own then you can keep from relying on others for comfort or energy.

Another way to learn to love yourself is learning how to say 'No'. We as humans are highly empathetic creatures who, a lot of the time, give our limited time and energy to others. And it's good to be there for people and to tend to their needs, but only if we're capable of doing so. If we're constantly looking out for and helping others, we never have any time to check in with ourselves. This can lead to a loss of self-identity, resentment towards others for not caring for you as much as you care for them, and physical and mental exhaustion. When we're constantly being there for others and never being there for ourselves, we are doing a disservice to the person we're around the most.

It's important to learn how to say no to others when you simply don't have the time or energy to help them. It's also important to say no when you need time to yourself. It will feel uncomfortable at first especially if this is something you've never done before, but the long-term benefits are great. You'll be much better at setting boundaries that show that you deserve and expect respect, you'll learn how to be assertive, and you'll put more value on your personal time.

Learning to love yourself also means learning your strengths and weaknesses and responding to them accordingly. We all have certain things that we're better at than others, and we also have those skills and traits that are admittedly weaker than others. This is what makes us uniquely human. However, distractions and self-doubt get in the way of us fully understanding and utilizing these strengths. Take the time now to consider what you feel like you're good at, and then ask yourself why you think so. Can you point to any accomplishments that you have to back up that strength? Have you ever been complimented about something multiple times? What do you find easy that others might find difficult? Let your gifts complement your self-image, allow them to be a part of the painting you're creating of yourself.

Accept that there are also things you aren't good at so that you remain humble. Loving yourself does not mean thinking that you're better than everybody. There is still a level of humility that you must have in self-love. Allow yourself to talk about your weaknesses, in a loving manner, and accept that having those flaws are okay. It's okay not to be perfect. Now if those weaknesses can be easily worked on and that's what you want to do, then that's okay too. But the first step before improving those weaknesses is acknowledging them.

And finally, learn to love yourself by learning how to forgive yourself. This has much to do with the previous point about weaknesses but also includes past, present, and future mistakes. Cringing over poor choices you've made is a sure sign of your growth as a person, so it's important to reflect on these times. But it's also important to tell yourself that you're better than you were that day and to learn to move on from the past. Holding on to your mistakes will hinder any forward growth, so remind yourself that you did the best you could and that you know better now.

Before we move on, I would love to mention that this is my very first book and I am so happy and grateful to be sharing it with you and an honest review would be highly appreciated.

Chapter Five

What's Eating You?

Stress.

It's a powerful thing.
Even looking at the word can make you *feel* stressed.

Stressors in our lives can make us feel like things are out of control, which can result in you looking for ways whether good or bad to take control of your life again. Being in a stressful situation or around stressful people makes us feel uncomfortable and frustrated, lowering our inhibitions and making us more inclined to do something impulsive. Too much stress in our lives affects us inside and out, it can cause our skin to break out in pimples and hives, put unnecessary strain on our cardiovascular system, and is one of the leading causes of depression and anxiety.

Stress Eating

Hippocrates once said to, 'let food be thy medicine, and medicine be thy food'. And there is great truth in that. Food is certainly meant to be a healing presence, but not in the way that stress allows it to. Stress is a powerful trigger, especially when it comes to eating; food intake suffers from the same level of severity as other functions and aspects of our lives. Stress on the body and mind has been linked to an increase in snacking on sweets and foods high in fat, regardless of hunger levels and the restraint they have towards their diet. It becomes almost an excuse to eat, really, when we're faced with a difficult situation and we either haven't processed it or don't want to. Ice cream is stereotypically linked with breakups, happy hour at bars and restaurants is right around the end of a typical workday, and we're prone to reaching for sugar and caffeine to get us through the rest of our day. This link between stress and food comes with a familiar term: stress eating.

Stress eating, or its other name 'emotional eating', doesn't do well with what we want to accomplish in this book. Stress strips the enjoyment of food, turning it into a solitary source of comfort, a coping mechanism, or a distraction from your problems. It contrasts with mindfulness and its practices, keeping us in our heads and out of the moment which will cause us to act more on our impulses. And those impulses can cause us to overeat and ruin carefully planned eating habits.

And of course, stress eating has nothing to do with being hungry. Stress is already linked to addiction and addiction relapse, so its presence around food causes it to function as a dangerous catalyst. This is because stress causes sensory overload which lowers resistance and inhibitions, causing people to relapse or reach for familiar vices much easier than they would before. One of those vices can be an unhealthy food intake.

And there are certain foods we gravitate towards more when we're stressed. Studies have shown that this is due to stress raising our cortisol levels, a chemical that allows us to make informed decisions when the body is on high alert.

This, in turn, leads to an increase in our insulin levels. It's why foods that are high in fat, sugar, and salt are much more appealing when we're stressed. Examples of these foods are cookies, chocolate bars, chips, and fries.

Stress eating is a dangerous enemy for our goal of a healthy mindset towards food. Fortunately for you, stress eating is not a life sentence. It's avoidable and reversible, and just as accessible as general stress relief is. But before we begin talking about certain methods to help with stress eating, it's important to ask yourself questions to see if you really are afflicted with stress eating.

Chances are, however, if you think that you're indulging in stress eating then you most likely are.

Do you eat when confronted with an uncomfortable situation even if you aren't hungry? Do you find yourself craving certain foods during certain situations or when you're feeling certain emotions? Do you eat when you feel like there's nothing else to do or when you're avoiding doing something? Does it feel like something is weighing you down and keeping you from living your best life?

A 'yes' to any of these questions can point to a problem with stress eating. And if you want help in kicking this unhelpful habit, then these tips will be very useful to you.

How To Manage Stress

One way to stop stress eating is learning how to manage the overall stress in your life. Learning how to deal with stress is useful in aiding your body and mind, helping you make more informed decisions on things such as what and when to eat. And fortunately, these tips don't require any special equipment nor are they time-consuming. These can be done during a stressful situation to keep yourself stable, or beforehand to bring yourself to a stress-free attitude throughout your day.

There are two key ways to deal with persistent stress: breathing and moving. These are two actions that we do subconsciously (much more so with breathing), but not something we usually do deliberately. Breathing has been touched on in this book as a supporting tool, but here with stress is where it's particularly useful because it helps release tension and ease our thoughts back into manageable levels. It is a quick way to relax our body and mind.

The specific kind of breathing that we want to focus on is done from the belly rather than up in the chest area like we're mostly used to, this is a practice known as breathing from your diaphragm and it's popular among singers and athletes. Place your hands around your navel or belly button and breathe while imagining your stomach filling up like a balloon. As your belly expands, your hands should no longer be touching, and as you exhale imagine that you're breathing out all the stress and anxiety you have through a long, slow breath. A simple way to ensure that you're taking long deep breaths is to count to four with each process. This means breathing in for four counts, holding in your breath for four counts, exhaling for four counts, and holding again for another four counts.

What about moving? *Is there a specific way that we should be moving to get rid of stress?* No, there isn't. Stress typically triggers our fight or flight response anyway, and so our body *wants* to move and react. If you're sitting down, the movement can be something as simple as pushing your shoulders down or standing up and walking around for a minute. Physical activity has been proven to bring your body back to homeostasis or a stable condition, and rigorous physical activity such as exercise especially helps because it releases endorphins and dopamine that can counter stress and increase productivity and concentration.

How To Stop Stress Eating

There are also things you can do to help specifically with stress eating. Remember that stress eating is a response from your mind and not from your stomach, which you'll see in these next few tips. That doesn't mean, however, that there aren't things we can change about what we eat. So we'll be attacking stress eating on two fronts: reshaping our mind and thought processes and introducing things in our diet that can ease stress and help our bodies in relaxing.

We'll start with talking about what you can put in your body that will help with stress eating and general wellness. Tea is a particularly effective stress-reliever due to its medicinal qualities, especially chamomile tea. This kind of tea has been used throughout history as a natural stress reliever due to its ability to relax the muscles, lower cortisol levels, and even has sedative qualities to help with a good night's sleep. Berries are also known to help with stress due to their antioxidants that help with inflammation and protect neural processes, and their Vitamin C content which helps in regulating cortisol and blood pressure levels. Another treat rich in antioxidants is dark chocolate, specifically those with barely any added sugar and a cocoa content level of seventy percent or higher. Fatty fish like salmon and tuna are rich in Omega-3 fatty acids that have been proven to help with a healthy brain and mind and protection against heart diseases and lowering blood pressure. And finally, shellfish such as oysters and clams relieve stress due to the amount of Vitamin B, magnesium, and taurine they have. Taurine is especially useful because it's an amino acid needed to create dopamine. Meanwhile,

Vitamin B helps with memory and relieves depression and anxiety symptoms, and magnesium helps us 'de-escalate' and fight stress.

When it comes to tackling stress via our minds, it's all about observation and prevention. First of all, you want to know what your stressors are, which means figuring out what in your life causes you such high, unnecessary levels of stress that you react through unhealthy ways like overeating or snacking to avoid said stressor. Before you go to eat, ask yourself the previous question of whether you're eating because you're hungry or if you're dealing with something? If it's the latter, it's important to make note of what made you feel the way you're feeling through a journal. Understanding where the source of your stress is coming from (for example, a rough relationship or unhealthy working conditions) can help you in dealing with those triggers. Once you identify your stressors, get rid of the foods you gravitate to when triggered or at least make them difficult to obtain. Especially if said foods are high in fat, salt, or sugar, which are easy to overindulge on. Afterward, try out the general stress-relief activities above like taking breaths or going on a walk, other activities you can try include drinking water or simply talking your problem out with someone.

Stress will not break you, or rather it shouldn't. You are stronger than what your mind perceives. Take extra care to relieve stress in your life because it will not only benefit your eating habits but will also benefit your mind and soul.

Chapter Six

Do You Eat To Live Or Live To Eat?

Stop right here for a moment and consider the title of this chapter. Without knowing anything about this chapter, what does this question mean to you? What kinds of emotions or memories does it bring up? Do you feel confident answering this or are you refraining until you have more information? In any case, this is not a trick question. There is one simple answer that I can't wait to discuss with you.

We need to be careful of the food we choose to consume regularly. While food is indeed a wonderful blessing, our lives are an even bigger blessing and we should prioritize that by choosing to eat foods that prolong and enrich our lives. This also means reducing our intake of junk foods, especially those high in saturated fat and salt content, sugary treats, and also certain dairy products. The problem is that we live in a world where these types of foods feel the most abundant and so we gravitate towards those foods quicker than healthier alternatives. Not only that, we prefer these foods more because they produce dopamine, which helps us feel happier, fulfilled, and leading us down a path of addiction due to wanting more of these feelings.

Because of this, people have stopped eating to live, and have begun living to eat. And it's this shift that is killing us from the inside out.

The rise in popularity and availability of fast-food restaurants is a direct link to the increase in saturated fat, salt, sugar, and dairy products. Low prices for large meals are a major selling point, especially for young people. Advertisements centered around food also heavily promote these kinds of foods, but we'll talk about that in a later chapter. And in places for entertainment, these are the main food choices that you can choose from while you're enjoying yourself. Another leading cause of the higher intake of these kinds of foods is the fact that meat and milk are some of the largest food staples of the Western world. And while delicious, these flavorful foods are full of fatal flaws.

Foods filled with saturated fat (especially those fried in unhealthy oils such as canola and corn) are one of the key contributors to heart disease due to an increase in cholesterol and lack of antioxidants. Dairy products are inherently harmful to the body, not only aiding the rise in lactose intolerance, but also playing a leading factor in coronary heart disease. A higher intake of salt can also do a number to your cholesterol, but it is also a leading factor in strokes and stomach cancer. And eating too much sugar puts you at risk for diabetes and other blood-related diseases.

While these facts might shock you, it should come as a bigger surprise to know just how unavoidable these foods are. Fast-food restaurants have burgers, fries, sandwiches, sodas, and several dessert options that give you maximum freedom over your spending power and also your food intake. But even if you're not big on fast food, there are still foods in our everyday lives that will be high in these harmful chemicals.

Innocent pastries at the local grocery store are actually full of sugars and preservatives, fruit juices are more sugar than they are fruit, diet sodas that applaud themselves for having zero calories are still full of harmful chemicals, salad dressings are loaded with oils and unhealthy fats, and white bread is low in fiber and surprisingly high in sugar. There are unhealthy food choices all around us, some more hidden than others, which is why it's so important that you choose foods that say that you eat to live.

Eating to Live

First of all, we must remind ourselves that we are not meant to cut foods completely out of our diets (if we aren't addicted to them) because that will cause them to be much more enticing. All food is good, even the unhealthiest foods still provide enjoyment for us because of the previously mentioned dopamine they develop for us. And fast food is nice once in a while when you don't feel like cooking or you need something quick (hence the name). It's only when we eat them far too regularly that things become a problem. This is why we say to eat everything in moderation because too much of anything can be bad for you.

There are, however, foods you can eat that are life-enriching, meant to heal you internally and sometimes externally, and allow you to easily choose to live. Simply put, there are foods out there that give life. Some of these might seem obvious, some of them might surprise you, but all of these foods are guaranteed to have multiple benefits in the form of vitamins and minerals that will aid your body and mind.

Foods That Help You Choose Life

We've already talked about how chamomile tea is great for relieving stress and for promoting a good night's sleep, but there are other kinds of teas that have benefits just as amazing. Green and black teas are full of antioxidants that promote long life due to their ability to prevent chronic diseases and strengthen your immune system. Plus, they're a healthier source of caffeine. Peppermint tea does well in relieving digestive issues and so it's useful for those with stomach pain, nausea, and irritable bowel syndrome. And sage tea helps greatly with the mind. Studies have shown that sage is useful in helping with cognitive functions, especially in regards to memory, and overall mood.

Fruits and vegetables are commonly known to be good for you due to the nutritious value infused into them. All fruits and vegetables are full of certain vitamins and minerals, are convenient snacks when you're craving something sweet or filling, and when prepared correctly they can be very flavorful and delicious. Certain fruits and vegetables, however, have individual benefits you might not know about. Apples have pectin, which is a fiber that helps with digestion and overall gut health. Bananas are high in potassium and when they're ripe, they're a great source of carbs. Avocados differ from other fruits. They are low on sugar and high on healthy fats. Kiwis are also a great source of fiber and potassium, but they're also rich in carotenoids which help with eye health. Spinach and other dark leafy green vegetables have antioxidants that reduce the risk of cancer. Broccoli is another vegetable effective against cancer along with helping ease stress on the heart. Sweet potato is, as the name implies, a rare sweet-tasting vegetable that is also a great source of fiber and protein and less starchy than its regular potato counterpart. Garlic has benefits outside of a delicious seasoning for other foods, its main ingredient allows it to be perfect for lowering cholesterol and regulating blood sugar.

Dark chocolate has amazing health benefits when you get into the seventy to eighty-five percent of cocoa levels. Not only is it also rich in antioxidants, but it's full of minerals such as magnesium, iron, and especially fiber. Magnesium is known as a natural pain reliever, which is why it's popular for women experiencing period cramps. It relaxes the arteries which produce a healthier blood flow and a small decrease in blood pressure. And though it still has sugar, it still has much less than chocolates with lower percentages of cocoa. This means that the darker chocolate you eat, the more you acclimate to that level of sweetness, which means other chocolates and desserts will be too sweet for you and you'll eat less of them.

Not all frying oil is bad for you. Monounsaturated oils such as canola, peanut, and olive oil not only provide a nice flavor to your fried foods, but they also have certain health benefits due. Their monounsaturated nature means they're liquid at room temperature and only start to harden as they cool, and its healthier nature gives your body its necessary amounts of fat while also lowering your risk for heart disease and cholesterol levels. Olive oil is especially beneficial. It contains antioxidants, Vitamins E and K, and can help protect against strokes and heart disease. Extra virgin olive oil is one of the main staples of a Mediterranean diet.

And finally, we look at the healthier options for meat. Burgers, steaks, and other kinds of red meat might be great sources of protein, they also put you at higher risks of diabetes and can-do major damage to your heart over time. Healthier options for meat are out there, ones that are leaner and just as delicious. Thinning out your steak choice can be helpful as well. Instead of going for the large ribs or T-bones, try sirloin steak instead. It's still a great source of protein and you get all the flavor without as much saturated fat. Take a chance on rotisserie chicken as well. It's already cooked and seasoned for you, and since chicken is a leaner white meat, it won't harm your cholesterol levels. Fish is already a food we've talked about in regards to relieving stress, but canned fish also has great benefits if you're looking for something a little more convenient. They're still filled with Omega-3 fatty acids and if they're canned in water or olive oil, you don't need to worry about needlessly added sodium.

Hopefully, the chapter's title makes much more sense to you. Choose to live and let the food fuel that, don't let food dictate how you live, or else you won't live for too long. Giving these foods a chance means giving yourself a chance. But what if you feel this temptation to skip this chapter's lessons? What if you feel a strong aversion towards the suggestions placed here? If you are full of these kinds of questions, then the next chapter will be greatly beneficial for you.

Chapter Seven

Train Your Mind To Love Healthy Eating

Now it's one thing to list all these healthy foods, it's another thing to actually include them in your diet. If these foods are a regular food group for you, then congratulations! You are ahead of the curve. But what about those of you who are just now considering the prospect of eating healthier? What about those of you who have tried the healthy eating lifestyle before but fell out for one reason or another? What about those of you who gag at the idea of eating a vegetable?

We set a judge-free zone in this book. Wherever you are in your health journey is just fine, it's all about forward movement. It's all about making progress. And getting used to healthy eating can be a hard mental block for you, which is okay and normal.

There is still a lot of hope for you, and you can progress just as much as everyone else. It just takes a little bit of mental adjustment. It means that you need to train your mind to love healthy eating.

Mental Blocks

There are several reasons that you might feel more averse to eating healthier. For some, it's a medical reason like you're allergic to a certain food. For others, it's a texture issue. They don't like how the food feels or tastes no matter how well they're prepared. These are the usual suspects, but when it's not your body keeping you away from these foods, then it's your mind. Mental blocks are a representation of being unable to remember something or to perform an action. These are regular occurrences that stem from past memories or a subconscious lineup of questions that cause you to be anxious enough to avoid doing something. In this case, these mental blocks are keeping you from trying healthier food choices. The sight of broccoli repulses you, eating an apple feels like an hour-long task, and you'd rather starve than eat a salad.

The mental block might be from a greater preference for other foods to the point of addiction. You *could* eat healthier and reach for fruits as a snack, but a chocolate bar sounds so much better. You can at least eat dark chocolate to get the health benefits from it, but your hand always hovers over the milk chocolate bars instead. You like snacks and junk food too much to eat healthier, but on the bright side, this mental block is reversible. Getting hooked on these foods is not a life sentence.

The mental block might come from temptation. Maybe you've tried committing to healthy eating, but you always find yourself reaching back to your vices. This can make you feel ashamed and result in a downward spiral that takes you back to where you started. While temptation can be a strong motivator, it's also a mental block that can be broken.

The mental block can be from a distorted body image. You might have stopped taking care of yourself or have neglected it for a while, telling yourself that you're at a healthy weight and that nothing needs to change. While there is nothing wrong with being confident in the body that you're in, blind confidence can lead to arrogance. And that means you feel yourself above changes to your lifestyle and health because you think that you're the best that you already are. But have you truly taken a look in the mirror and liked what you saw? Or are you just telling yourself that? Feeling good about your body doesn't mean you're allowed to stop taking care of it. A healthy body will make you more confident than you've ever been because it was built from your hard work and self-awareness that leaves you humble yet satisfied.

The mental block could be for the complete opposite problem. Maybe you have zero confidence and have been unhappy with your body for such a long time that you've given up on yourself. Maybe you've stopped looking in the mirror not because you like what you see but because you're deeply ashamed. Loving yourself is hard, but the most permanent love and happiness comes from ourselves. If this is your mental block, I strongly suggest re-reading the chapter on learning how to love yourself. You're worth so much more than you think, and you deserve to feel confident in yourself.

Finally, the mental block can stem from a fear of failure. There are some of us who are afraid of failing or losing, and so we avoid situations where that's too strong of an outcome. This might stem from a poor self-image, bad experiences in the past, or a harsh upbringing. Whatever the case may be, it's important to realize that you can still find a silver lining in failure. You learn how to be better, are more confident the next time around, and it instills a sense of humility in you that will help you stay on track with whatever you're doing.

Especially when it comes to a change in diet. Remember that learning how to eat healthier is not a competition. The only person you should be comparing yourself to is the person you were yesterday. If you're tempted to go back to vices, lower the restrictions on your diet so you don't spiral down into shame. Remember to stay grounded and take long, hard looks at yourself as a reminder of the body you're working for. And remember that you deserve happiness in any way that it's attainable for you.

Retraining Your Brain

Once you've identified the mental block(s) that could hinder your progress, it's time to retrain your brain so that your perspective on healthy foods can change. Remember that you're not alone in this fight. People throughout the day are always craving sugar, caffeine, and foods high in fat, but we weren't born with this kind of inhibition. We were conditioned throughout our entire lives to prefer these foods more to healthier options because they're the most readily available options. It's usually not that we find healthier foods to be gross tasting, it's more because we find non-healthy foods to be the tastier option.

Fortunately, it's not that hard to retrain your brain into preferring or at least including healthier foods in your diet. There's going to be some hesitation, not just from the mental blocks, but also because we live in a world where instant gratification is the norm and all-or-nothing thinking dominates our lives. We want results now and we see things in black-and-white.

Know that even though this ride is much easier than you believe it to be, it will still be long and require dedicated time. You won't see results right away, especially if you fall into that all-or-nothing attitude and try to switch up your entire diet in one day. If you think the plan to retrain your brain involves waking up tomorrow so you can run a mile even though you haven't done any running since high school, and then eating a large plate of salad afterward, then think again.

We start with small changes and we give ourselves time to see the results.

For starters, you want to limit the unhealthy cravings around you by getting rid of easily accessible foods that you can't seem to get enough of. Any addiction is bad, and you don't want to spend half your day justifying unnecessary snacking. This is an exercise in willpower that will get easier in time. Remember, however, to not cut foods out of your diet entirely because it could help develop a negative mindset around food. Junk food is fine on occasion, especially if you're able to regulate yourself, but for general snacking it's best to have healthier alternatives around.

Avoid the all-or-nothing by giving yourself the grace of including the healthy foods in your diet that you want rather than forcing yourself to eat all the healthy options. Forcing yourself to eat foods just because they're healthy will cause you to hate those certain foods, which will make you more inclined to go back to your old eating habits. Welcome the foods that you like and dismiss the ones you don't. If you like the taste of dark leafy greens but can't stand the taste of ginger or sweet potatoes, then just add the greens to your diet. If you love berries but don't like the crunch and taste of apples, then stick to berries. If you can't stand brown rice but whole-wheat pasta is calling your name, then go with the pasta. One is better than zero, adding a couple of healthy food options to your permanent diet is better than trying to include all of them and subsequently giving up on all of them.

Make water a greater part of your diet. While the amount of water that people need every day will vary due to their age, location, and their activity level, studies have shown that people just aren't drinking enough water. We tend to go for energy drinks and caffeine so that we can function throughout the day when water can in fact give us that needed energy as well. Not only that, but water also aids digestion, lowers your body temperature if you are too warm, regulates your heartbeat, and balances your electrolyte levels. It can also get rid of sporadic hunger pangs; one drink of water can keep you from snacking long enough to have a regular-sized meal.

An all-or-nothing line of thinking that is ingrained into a lot of us is this idea that we *need* to finish everything on our plate. We touched on this earlier in the book, and it bears repeating that the pressure to have clean plates at the end of the meal disregards the mindset of eating until you feel full. You need to tell yourself that it's okay not to eat everything on your plate, that if you feel full then you're full. You can save the rest of the food as leftovers or you can just throw it away. It might seem wasteful to throw the food away, but it's just as wasteful to eat it when you're not hungry. Eating more than you should will distort your idea of fullness while eating only what you can finish will allow you to better understand your limits.

And when you're choosing the healthier option, remember exactly *why* it's healthy. Sometimes while you're eating a salad or choosing vegetables as a side, you'll find yourself regretting your decision knowing you could have had fries instead. But it's not just about flavor when it comes to healthy foods. They're meant to help you live longer, happier lives that you're able to enjoy. They enrich both your body and mind. They will benefit you in the long run so that when you *do* eat fries, you're not overindulging or harming your insides. Plus, healthy food prepared correctly can be just as flavorful as whatever you're craving. Refer back to the last chapter if you need a refresher on what kind of health benefits your food choices will give you.

This chapter might have been the most involved chapter of them all. We're not only asking you to retrain your mind, but to also build off the information from a previous chapter and take deliberate steps in changing your diet. Don't be discouraged, you've gotten this far and I know that you can go further. We have one more topic to talk about, one final influential factor on your chances at living a healthier life. And it might not be a factor that you're expecting.

Chapter Eight

Listen To Your Body, Not the TV

We've talked a lot about the internal factors that go into changing the way we view food, hunger, and our bodies. What we haven't touched on that much are the external factors that influence as well. Those we choose to spend our time with will influence us with their own eating habits and viewpoint on food, our upbringing definitely plays a major part in certain mindsets we bring to the table, and the availability of certain foods will affect the kind of nutrition we have access to.

But there's one powerful influential factor that twists our viewpoint more than all the others: media. What we see on billboards and marketing, the shows and movies that we watch, and declarations by public figures play a surprisingly large part in our mindset toward food. This chapter will expose the methods in which the media does this and what we can do to keep from being over-influenced by things outside of our own minds.

Media's Influence on Food Intake

What are we talking about when we say media? What does the media entail? Media can be classified as any means of mass communication such as television shows, billboards, and the Internet. It is nearly impossible not to be influenced by the media in some way, shape, or form because we consume it in multiple ways throughout our everyday lives. Nowadays, we have much more of a choice as to what we consume, but the point remains that what we view affects how we feel and what we do. This is especially true when it comes to food and our bodies. There are two primary ways that the media influences our food intake: the marketing for certain products, and the roles that TV, movie, and social media play in promoting the 'ideal' body image. We will look at these methods one by one to show how each element corresponds to our mindsets and attitudes, while also creating a link between what we watch and what we eat.

Food Marketing

The point of food marketing is to push the sales of one product over another. Marketing can be something subliminal like a character in a movie drinking a certain beer, or it can be right in your face like a billboard using flashy words and eye-catching details. They'll partner with currently popular figures to promote their foods, constantly promote deals so that you feel like you're getting a better deal by buying more food than you initially wanted to. Companies use their knowledge of cravings and trends throughout the year so that they know what to market and when, examples of this include the rise in candy sales during Halloween and the extensive food and drink commercials during events like the Super Bowl where they know a large number of consumers will be watching TV.

Fast food restaurants are especially guilty of marketing. In an era where standing out is difficult yet crucial for businesses *and* people, fast food chains have to constantly find new ways to market themselves above their competitors. They implement certain strategies through their commercials, print advertisements, customer service, and online presence. One such method is the head-to-head approach, where they stack their product against their competitors, touting advantages such as the size of their product, the freshness of their ingredients, and the amount of food you can get for cheaper prices. Another more recent method is to implement 'loyalty rewards' for returning customers. By signing up for a rewards program or by downloading their app, customers can order their food beforehand while also receiving 'points' for being a loyal customer that can go toward discounts or free food. Another very effective method that they use is to play on our inherent 'fear of missing out' by only making certain foods available for a limited time. Since they aren't on the regular, permanent menu, you want to try it out before it's going on so that you stay up to date on the newer, trendier foods that people are talking about.

The effect that this has on consumers (in every sense of the word) is subtle but frightening. Studies have found a positive correlation between food advertising and automatic snacking. Even when people aren't hungry, the sight of food (especially unhealthy food) makes them more inclined to reach for the snacks and eat something. The sights and sounds, combined with the other predatory marketing tactics, trigger something in people's minds that make them want what they see on TV or at least something similar. That unneeded snacking and eating when not hungry obviously leads to major weight gain, and a subtle inclination towards these unhealthier foods.

The Ideal Body Image

In recent decades and especially throughout the 21st century, the media has always praised and preferred a slender body type. The people on TV and in movies are tall and skinny, with the women having nice curves and a tight frame and the men having strong, muscular builds. Up until recently, teenagers in shows and movies were portrayed by actors in their twenties. On social media, you're more likely to get likes and comments if you're fit and attractive, with pictures depicting you living a perfect, free life. And teenagers (the main demographic) look at their own lives and bodies with disdain, not yet understanding that these moments are fabricated and the lighting and angles in the picture are helping to create the illusion of perfection. Women are bombarded with skincare and weight loss ads, men get muscle-building and fitness ads. It's rare if you find clothing and underwear advertisements with plus-sized models, and even rarer to find advertisements where the models aren't wearing makeup.

The message is clear: there is only one acceptable body image for men and women. And chances are you don't fit it.

While we're much more aware of these trends than we have been in the past, and companies and people are making strides to promote natural beauty and body positivity, the effects from this message will be felt for a very long-time. Filters that alter your body and face are very popular on social media because people (especially young ones) are comparing themselves to the people on their feed and are changing themselves to look just like them. Teas and shakes that promote rapid weight loss are still being sold and advertised. Plus-sized and 'natural' models are still a rarity, further feeding into the illusion that you're not ideal. Things still need to change for the better.

Young women are especially susceptible to the kind of harm media places on their body image. Studies have shown that most young girls aged nine to fourteen feel like it's important that they're just as thin as the women they see on TV and movies, and they were found to be more susceptible to indulge in unhealthy methods of weight loss like purging and skipping meals. A lot of these girls believe that they're overweight even if they're in the normal weight range of people their age.

Breaking the Illusion

It's important to first mention that these predatory media tactics are much less prevalent than they were even just a decade ago thanks to advancements in communication technology and younger people being taken much more seriously. With the ability to address a massive amount of people in a short amount of time, companies are quickly chastised when they run advertisements that promote unhealthy body images and eating habits. Celebrities, musicians, and other kinds of public figures are using their platform to remind people to love their bodies and are teaching how important it is to take care of them through proper nutrition and exercise. Modeling agencies are beginning to impose proper weight limits so that models need to be *above* a certain weight limit instead of below it in order to curb the rise in eating disorders and body dysmorphia. And recent food trends have shown a rise in more organic eating, with more people reaching for non-processed foods and learning how to cook than ever before.

Things are better than they used to be, external influences are becoming much less harmful. But there is still work that needs to be done internally if we want to fully break from the media's influence on us. The most important thing that needs to be done is that we need to have a stronger sense of media literacy. What this means is that we need to identify all different kinds of media and the messages they're trying to send. It means understanding when we're being advertised to and what the advertisement wants us to believe. It's investigating behind-the-scenes of movies and TV shows to see how accurate the actors are in portraying the characters they need to be, and knowing just how much air brushing, makeup, and a rigorous fitness plan can drastically change someone's look. It's knowing how to peel the curtain back on social media posts to see what filters are being used on the faces and bodies, figuring out whether the shots are posed or candid, and knowing the importance of angles, lighting, and posture are.

Once we're aware of just *how* the media creates these images, we begin to realize all the work it takes to make something look perfectly natural while also realizing that *perfectly* natural doesn't exist the way we're seeing it. Also, take great care in thinking carefully over who you are drawn to more, consider your favorite actors, social media influencers, and even video game characters, seeing if they have anything in common. While it's nice to fantasize and even dress up as your favorites during appropriate occasions, be careful that you're not trying to emulate everything about them. Not just how they look, but also how they behave.

The only way to know how perfectly natural looks is to look in the mirror. What you see is what's real, unfabricated, and a better image of a body as it's regularly meant to be.

Which brings us to our second important way to break the media's illusion over body image; We need to learn how to listen to our bodies and be comfortable with ourselves. We've talked about the importance of both of these, but the advice bears repeating. Advertisements will tell us when we should eat and what we're hungry for, but our stomach is the one we should be listening to. Only eat when you're hungry, and stop eating when you're full. Don't constantly go for junk food and fast food when healthier options will fill you up even more, but don't cut them out entirely either so they aren't too tempting. Be loyal to your body and needs, not to a fast-food chain and their phone app.

Be comfortable in your own skin and what you see in the mirror. Yes, it's okay to want to change things about yourselves, but don't do it because of something or someone you saw on the television screen or on your phone. Change what you want because you want to be healthier, more confident, and the best person you can possibly be. The only person that you are in competition with is yourself, don't let outside forces dictate the steps you take in your journey.

Listen to what your body is telling you, not what the TV says. Not what the computer says. Not what your phone says. Don't let anyone or anything else dictate how you should view yourself or change the way you think. You'll always know yourself better than anyone else.

Chapter Nine

Applying Everything

Now, dear reader, we have reached the end of our journey together. The seeds you planted along this road will bear great fruit for you in the near and distant future. Remember that this was not meant to be a shameful look at everything you were doing wrong with your life, but rather a celebratory view of the life you now get to live. Food is a great provider and a universal communicator; it brings people together and teaches us things we never would have learned on our own. We bathed our food in salt to preserve it, and now we have refrigerators that do that for us. Yeasts and bacteria come together to somehow create things such as beer, cheese, yogurt, and bread. And most recently, we have found a way to use plant-based products to make meat-tasting products. Food is a testament to progress and innovation.

The more we learn about food, the more we should appreciate just how much it does for us. Your appreciation for food can only grow from here with what you have learned, and what you've learned will make you a stronger and more capable person able to tackle any challenge. Not just with food, but also with hunger and your body, and the several factors that go into why we eat. Don't let these words fall to the wayside. Read through this book more than once, finding details that you may have missed, and applying all the lessons through each chapter.

Remember to keep your relationship with food in check, knowing that a bad relationship with food is centered around guilt, resentment, and over-control and that a good relationship with food is centered around joy for the opportunity to eat. Take the steps necessary in building a good relationship to heart. Don't exclude foods, give yourself unconditional permission to eat whatever you want to, but ensure that you're only eating when hungry and stopping when full.

Remember how important it is to learn mindful eating, and learning to differentiate it from mindless eating. Mindless eating is also known as distracted eating, it's eating when you're not hungry and not in the right headspace to enjoy the food that you're having. Consider the steps you need to take to learn mindful eating and how deceptively easy it is to start. Get rid of distractions while eating, and eat slowly so that you can savor the food and its flavors.

Remember how easy it is to start overeating and not feel like you can stop. Look at the reasons someone might overeat and see if they fit your predicament. Know that there are twenty-one other ways to help combat overeating aside from moderating your food intake. Are there certain methods or tips that you feel more confident doing over others?

Remember to draw a distinct line between what it means to hate yourself or love yourself, and choose the side where you love yourself. Betterment spurred on by self-hate will inevitably go bad and you'll never think that you're enough. It might seem scary to take that leap and learn how to love yourself, especially if you're not used to working on yourself, but know that you're deserving of love just as much as the ones you give love to. And if you're not going to love yourself, who will? And don't forget that wanting to lose weight or eat healthier doesn't mean you hate your body, it means you love yourself enough to want to live a longer, healthier life.

Remember how damaging stress can be on our body and mind, and how easy it can creep up on you from the smallest of inconveniences to the largest of life-changers. Understand how crippling stress can be, how it can raise our blood pressure, make us more susceptible to anxiety and depression, and make us more inclined to snack and overeat on unhealthy foods. Give yourself the gift of peace through the stress-relief activities along with implementing the foods and drinks into your diet that can help you overcome stress such as chamomile tea, berries, and fatty fish.

Remember that you should choose to eat foods that are life-giving rather than living for foods that give you temporary sustenance. Understand the dangers of the food we typically gravitate towards like the ones high in saturated fats, salt, and sugar, and see the link between those and an increase in heart disease, diabetes, and other ailments that will kill you from the inside out. Understand the foods that will help us overcome these unhealthy eating habits like dark leafy greens, teas, and leaner meats.

Remember that while it is fairly easy to introduce healthier foods into your diet, it's difficult to train your brain to accept these inclusions. Be cognizant of the mental blocks that might exist in your mind which could hinder your ability to accept these changes. Mental blocks such as addiction towards certain foods, a distorted body image, a fear of failure, or an all-or-nothing line of thinking. Have confidence in yourself to overcome these mental blocks while taking small, simple steps to introduce healthier foods into your diet. It doesn't take much, and it doesn't take a lot of grand gestures. Find the healthy foods that you like and permanently add them to your existing diet, be comfortable with leaving food on your plate when you're full and remind yourselves of just how much these foods are benefiting you inside and out.

Remember that there are external factors that have an influence on your eating habits, and that the biggest one is the media that we consume on a regular basis. Know the tricks that advertisements use to hook you into buying certain foods and pulling you towards certain fast-food places or restaurants. Be wary of product placements and understand that these food corporations only care about you buying their product. Identify and call out the unhealthy body standards that are all over TV, movies, and social media; notice that even now they continue to push this ideal body image that not many people can live up to. Understand that you shouldn't compare yourself to that image and become more media literate so that you know what messages the media is trying to tell you and how they're doing it.

Before we conclude, I want to leave you with a few more lessons that are meant to add onto what you've already learned. First of all, it's important for you to know how much of an impact that habits have in our daily lives. We all have unconscious, neutral habits such as how we get out of bed, how we brush our teeth, and how we put on our clothes. We also have good habits such as schedules for exercising or studying. And we also have bad habits such as overeating, nails biting, or grabbing a chocolate bar at the checkout aisle before you pay. You may have noticed that this book is meant to motivate you to learn and reinforce good habits and upheaving the bad ones. And it doesn't take that long for you to establish a habit provided that you continuously and deliberately commit to the action. It's much harder to break a habit, which is unfortunate for the bad habits that we need to break.

Take a day to be mindful of your actions and note what kind of things you do almost automatically, because that's a sign that it's a developed habit. Note the good ones and neutral ones, and separate them from the habits that aren't serving you. Commit to not only breaking these habits, but replacing them with better ones. For example, if you find yourself wanting to drink caffeine late in the day, replace that habit with a quick walk or a break from whatever environment you're in. Don't be discouraged if you find yourself slipping into these bad habits accidentally, that's the all-or-nothing mindset trying to shame you for not being better *now*. Understand that what you did to create that habit is what it will take to break it, and that with small steps, you'll eventually develop a healthier habit in its stead. It's the power of repetition combined with the power of habits at work, keep moving forward and don't give up on yourself.

Know that if you don't apply every single step in this book and take every piece of advice, it doesn't mean you're failing. Do what's best for you and your body. If that means taking some steps toward mindfulness and adding salmon to your diet, then that's fine. If you take everything to heart and plan to implement everything you've read, then that's fine too. There are many factors you need to consider when going through this book, things you need to accept about yourself so that you don't think you're doing things wrong. The methods you choose to undertake have to suit you, your thought patterns and your beliefs, your upbringing and how you were raised to consider food in your house. Was it in abundance? Was it scarce? Were your parents strict with what to eat and when? Or did they let you eat whatever and whenever?

Don't try and force yourself to do things that you aren't comfortable with, things that clash with your beliefs or biological makeup, things that you've tried and just didn't like doing. You know you better than anyone else, and what works for someone else may not work for you. This is *your* journey, *your* changing mindset, *your* body that's being worked on.

I cannot stress enough how important it is to stay hydrated and make water your main drink. If need be, you can add flavoring or get seltzer water, but rest assured water does so much good for your organs and your skin that it would be criminal for you not to drink it. Along with water, it's also highly important that you are getting a good night's sleep every night and taking naps when necessary. Your body and mind do a lot of recovery through sleep, and it's a proven remedy against stress and overthinking. No matter what is in your schedule, ensure that there is enough time for you to get the recommended seven to nine hours of sleep every night. Your body needs it, your mind needs it.

And last but certainly not least, it's important that you are kind, patient, and loving with yourself. You are a brave, wonderful, strong human being full of so much potential to be whatever you want to be. Every decision you make should be meant to serve and develop the person you were always meant to be, but before you get to that point you need to love yourself right where you are. Take the time every day to tell yourself that you are enough because you *so* are. You have always been enough and will continue to be enough as you go farther along this journey. Because there is no competition or comparison, there is just you and the work that you're putting in. You, dear reader, are worth so much and you need to believe that if you're ever going to be successful in being the best version of yourself. Learn to love yourself just as you are, embrace what you can't change about yourself such as your height, your beautiful eyes and other features that make you unique and stand out, and work on wherever there is room for improvement without ever comparing yourself to anyone out there.

Be confident in your abilities. You are wise enough to take away great lessons from this book and have an open mind to let at least one chapter or line resonate with you for the rest of your life. You have the strength and willpower to make good choices and develop good habits. You have the awareness to treat your body right by staying safe, hydrated, and well-rested. You are gracious enough to enjoy food as a gift above all else. And you have the chance now to better enjoy the other gifts afforded to you which can never be taken away: life and love.

You are brave, strong, loving, and capable of great things. Through your own power and the knowledge of this book, tomorrow you will wake up hungry for life.

Conclusion

You are what you eat. That phrase must mean

something entirely different to you now after what you've learned throughout this book. It could mean that you are the product of the food you choose to indulge in on a regular basis. It could mean that the quality of food you're putting into your body will dictate the life you live. It could also mean that what you crave food-wise can tell you more about what you crave in life.

Take one more moment to consider what that phrase means to you now that you've reached the end of this book. And then take a second to consider what food truly means to you now. For I know what it means to me.

Food is neither good nor bad, food is energy and is there to be enjoyed. It offers fuel and happiness to your mind and body and as long as you respect that body enough to give it a variety of foods on a daily basis, you will feel more organized, you will believe in yourself, you will feel balanced and in equilibrium inside and out.

There is one powerful affirmation I would like you to use often, "Every day in every way, life just keeps getting better and better." Because you now have a vision, your thoughts have changed, your mind now works for you and you're taking the action that shapes your new reality.

Do you still have an excuse for not eating healthy or not getting in shape? Because what I see is nothing but massive potential to achieve what you truly believe it's best for you and your lifestyle. And always remember, your mind loves compliments so by making a choice of constantly praising yourself for your newly healthy habits, how fabulous you look and most importantly how wonderful you feel, you will make sure you are on the right path going strong every single day.

Let's keep in touch, I would love to hear from you:

Facebook: Oana Piticar
Instagram: oanapiticar

Here's to the "full of life" you!
With much love,

Oana Piticar
2021

References

Beshara, M., Hutchinson, A. D., & Wilson, C. (2013). Does mindfulness matter? Everyday mindfulness, mindful eating and self-reported serving size of energy dense foods among a sample of South Australianadults. *Appetite*, *67*, 25–29. https://doi.org/10.1016/j.appet.2013.03.012

Bjarnadottir, A. (2019, June 19). *Mindful Eating 101 — A Beginner's Guide*. Healthline. https://www.healthline.com/nutrition/mindful-eating-guide#what-it-is

Cline, R. (2018). *Mindful vs. Mindless Eating: NCHPAD - Building Inclusive Communities*. National Center on Health, Physical Activity and Disability (NCHPAD). https://www.nchpad.org/1693/6799/Mindful~vs~~Mindless~Eating

Connolly, A. (2018, October 25). *12 Mental Blocks That Sabotage Diets*. Motivation Weight Management. https://motivation.ie/mental-weight/how-to-overcome-the-12-mental-blocks-that-can-sabotage-diets/

Davidson, K. (2020, December 3). *5 Tips for Developing a Better Relationship with Food*. Healthline.

https://www.healthline.com/nutrition/fixing-a-bad-relationship-with-food#tips

Groesz, L. M., McCoy, S., Carl, J., Saslow, L., Stewart, J., Adler, N., Laraia, B., & Epel, E. (2012). What is eating you? Stress and the drive to eat. *Appetite, 58*(2), 717–721. https://doi.org/10.1016/j.appet.2011.11.028

Healthy Set Go. (2021, April 21). *Top foods to relieve stress.* Allina Health. https://www.allinahealth.org/healthysetgo/nourish/top-foods-to-relieve-stress

Hurst, K. (2017, November 9). *How To Love Yourself And Be Confident With These 15 Self Love Tips.* The Law of Attraction. https://www.thelawofattraction.com/love-yourself/

Kubala, J. (2019, December 1). *23 Ways to Stop Overeating.* Healthline. https://www.healthline.com/nutrition/how-to-stop-overeating

Kyte, J. (2015, July 8). *Train Your Brain To Love Healthy Eating.* Woman and Home Magazine. https://www.womanandhome.com/health-and-wellbeing/train-your-brain-to-love-healthy-eating-111159/

Martin, S. (2018, February 10). *How to Love Yourself: 22 Simple Ideas.* Live Well with Sharon Martin. https://www.livewellwithsharonmartin.com/how-to-love-yourself/

Migala, J. (2019, June 10). *How to Use Moderation as a Weight-Loss Tool | Weight Loss | MyFitnessPal.* MyFitnessPal. https://blog.myfitnesspal.com/how-to-use-moderation-as-a-weight-loss-tool/

Morris, A. M., & Katzman, D. K. (2003). The impact of the media on eating disorders in children and adolescents. *Paediatrics & Child Health, 8*(5), 287–289.

https://www.ncbi.nlm.nih.gov/pmc/articles/PMC2792687/

Peer, M. (2012, February 9). *Junk Food | Marisa Peer | Weight Loss Hypnotherapy*. Marisa Peer. https://marisapeer.com/junk-food/

Peer, M. (2013, January 29). *How To Stop Overeating? Identify Which Type Of Eater You Are*. Marisa Peer. https://marisapeer.com/how-to-stop-overeating/

Peer, M. (2019a, April 16). *Coping with Stress - 10 Proven Stress Management Activities*. Marisa Peer. https://marisapeer.com/stress-management-activities/

Peer, M. (2019b, July 17). *How To Be Healthy - You are What You Eat, Think and Do*. Marisa Peer. https://marisapeer.com/how-to-be-healthy-you-are-what-you-eat-think-and-do/

Petre, A. (2019, April 11). *13 Science-Backed Tips to Stop Mindless Eating*. Healthline; Healthline Media. https://www.healthline.com/nutrition/13-tips-to-stop-mindless-eating

Richards, P. (2017, August 14). *How Does Media Impact Body Image and Eating Disorder Rates?* Center for Change. https://centerforchange.com/how-does-media-impact-body-image-and-eating-disorder-rates/

Scott, J. (2019). *How to Stop Eating When You're Not Hungry but Stressed*. Verywell Fit. https://www.verywellfit.com/what-is-emotional-eating-3495967

The Health Sciences Academy. (2014, October 15). *Can You Train Your Brain To Like Healthy Foods?* The Health Sciences Academy. https://thehealthsciencesacademy.org/health-tips/train-your-brain-to-like-healthy-foods/

TV Food Advertising Increases Snacking and Potential Weight Gain in Children and Adults. (2009, July 1).

YaleNews. https://news.yale.edu/2009/07/01/tv-food-advertising-increases-snacking-and-potential-weight-gain-children-and-adults#:~:text=TV%20Food%20Advertising%20Increases%20Snacking%20and%20Potential%20Weight%20Gain%20in%20Children%20and%20Adults

Weisburger, J. H. (2000). Eat to live, not live to eat. *Nutrition*, *16*(9), 767–773. https://doi.org/10.1016/s0899-9007(00)00400-7

Yau, Y. H. C., & Potenza, M. N. (2013). Stress and eating behaviors. *Minerva Endocrinologica*,*38*(3), 255–267. https://www.ncbi.nlm.nih.gov/pmc/articles/PMC4214609/